MW01519562

The Breathing Exercise Bible:
Relaxation and Meditation Techniques for Happiness and Healthy Living

By Anthony Anholt

Discover other fitness titles by Anthony Anholt

The Isometric Exercise Bible

The Bodyweight Exercise Bible

The Abdominal Exercise Bible

Jump Rope Workouts

Disclaimer

Table Of Contents

Why is Deep Breathing Important for Happiness and Healthy Living?

The body is like a piano, and happiness is like music. It is needful to have the instrument in good order. - Henry Ward Beecher

To social reformer and abolitionist Henry Ward Beecher, the key to life long happiness and healthy living was maintaining a sound mind and body. I agree with him. Right now take a moment and think of anything in your life that truly gives you a feeling of happiness and contentment. It could be your work, your family, or even various hobbies and pastimes. Now think about this. Whatever your passions are, how many of them can you enjoy if you are in poor health? You could be the richest man or woman on the planet, but what's the point if you're not healthy enough to enjoy it? Truly the foundation of a happy life, more than anything, is your health. As many fitness pioneers have pointed out, your wealth is your health. With it, the world is at your fingertips. Without it, you are lost.

And what is the foundation of a healthy body? Is it constantly working out to have toned muscles? Eating a proper diet? Getting enough sleep? Sure, all of these things are vital, but what is the one critical factor that trumps them all? What is the foundation upon which all of them rest? The modern health practitioner might have difficulty with this question, but old school health advocates knew the answer. To them the foundation of your health is your breath and proper breathing.

Both yoga and the martial arts put a tremendous amount of emphasis on the importance of breathing properly. In fact both the Chinese and Indians believed that we all possessed a "second skin" that existed just below the surface of our physical being. This skin was not a skin of flesh, however, but a skin of energy. When this energy skin is alive, vibrant and healthy so are we. Keeping our "second skins" vibrant and healthy is the primary purpose behind such concepts as "Pranayama" and "Chi Kung".

The importance of proper breathing was not unknown in the western world either. In the late 19th and early 20th century health advocates of all stripes put a tremendous amount of emphasis on the importance of deep breathing. To them how healthy you were on the inside was just as important as how you looked on the outside. Believe it or not there were actually schools dedicated to simply learning various breathing techniques.

In recent years however the importance of proper breathing as a foundation of good health has thankfully been making a comeback. Why? Due to the simple fact that the benefits gained from engaging in proper, deep, diaphragmatic breathing are enormous. Here is a list of just some of the benefits you can expect when you resolve to practice deep breathing:

- Increased lung power and stamina
- Slows the aging process
- Improves your circulation
- Increases your energy levels

- Aides in digestion and elimination
- Purges your body of toxins
- Turbo charges your metabolism
- Helps with weight loss and weight maintenance
- Reduces anxiety and stress
- Helps conditions such as insomnia and asthma
- Is an excellent form of mediation which helps with mental focus and creativity

And this is only a partial list.

I know that upon reading this you might be skeptical. How can proper breathing, an act most of us do without even thinking about, have such a great effect? To understand why we need to look at how breathing affects the body from two perspectives: the physical and the mental. Let's do that now.

Breathing and the Physical Body

Without health, life is not life; it is only a state of languor and suffering – Francois Rabelais

In order to understand why proper breathing is so vital in maintaining a healthy life it is helpful to examine the body as if it were a biological machine (which in fact, it is). Any machine you can think of, whether mechanical or biological, requires energy to run. What's more it needs the proper kind of energy, delivered in the proper way, in order to run well. A car, for example, is designed to mix a certain amount of gas with oxygen. When a spark is added a controlled explosion occurs which generates energy. It is this energy that turns the drive shaft and propels the car forward. What happens though if the car is fed poor fuel or if the oxygen and gas are mixed in less than their ideal proportions? You guessed it. The car will not perform well or may not even run at all.

When it comes to generating energy our bodies are not that different from a car. Our bodies produce energy by combining fuel (carbohydrates) and oxygen in the proper proportions. This mixture is then burned, just like a car, in order to produce life energy. The only real difference between the two is that your body burns its fuel at a much slower and lower temperature. What is important to remember though is just like a car if your body is fed poor food or air of poor quality, or if it is not mixed correctly, your body will run poorly as well. Whereas your car will stall you as a biological machine will likely feel drowsy, old and tired. What's even worse is that as you are burning your fuel inefficiently you will likely wind up storing more of it in the form of fat.

The second way that deep breathing promotes health is through the elimination of toxins from the body. It does this by expelling carbon dioxide and other waste products when you exhale, which most people understand. What most people don't understand however is that proper breathing is also critical to a properly functioning lymphatic system. What exactly is your lymphatic system? Think of it as the equivalent of your bodies sewage system. Your body uses lymph fluid, of which your body has four times as much as blood, to purge wastes from your system. In fact if it were to shut down for whatever reason you would literally poison yourself within 24 hours and die. What is different about your lymphatic system is that it has no pump to circulate fluid throughout the body. It is completely reliant on body movement and breathing to circulate. By helping to keep your lymphatic system working at peak efficiency is another reason that breathing properly is vital to good health.

Happiness, Breathing and the Mind

A healthy body is a guest-chamber for the soul; a sick body is a prison – Francis Bacon

Although only a small percentage of the population understand the relationship between proper breathing and a healthy body, even less understand the relationship between proper breathing and a healthy mind. The truth is that your breath is the road that connects your mind with your body. Consider this. When you are calm and relaxed so is your breath. On the other hand when you are stressed or panicked your breath typically becomes quicker and shallower. I've seen some yogi's, who are experts at breath control, seemingly be able to read minds by simply observing the person's breath.

What is interesting though is that the mind body connection is a two way street. If you are not aware of it your "monkey mind" tends to control your breathing. However when you are aware of this fact you can actually use your breath to calm your mind. Mental states involving stress, insomnia, anxiety, panic attacks and depression can all be greatly mitigated if not eliminated by learning to calm your mind by controlling your breath. Calm, slow deep breathing is the key.

How Do You Breathe Properly?

*The groundwork of all happiness is health –
James Leigh Hunt*

In order to understand why there are so many benefits to breathing properly we need to look at the process of breathing itself. The first thing to know is that the nose is designed to be the primary system by which we inhale and exhale breath for, unlike the mouth, it is designed to clean and prepare the air before it reaches our lungs. Here's how it does this.

When air first enters the nose it must first pass through nasal hair, which removes any fine particles that it may contain. The air then passes over three seashell like structures called turbinates. The turbinates job is to stir up the incoming air and force it to circulate over a much larger surface than would otherwise be the case. This helps to correct the air temperature (either heating it up or cooling it down) and humidity level so that it is ideally suited to enter the delicate lungs. In addition to this the interior of the nose is also coated with a constantly moving mucous membrane that is able to absorb dust, bacteria and viruses. Most people are only aware of this membrane when they are sick and the mucous runs out of the nose. In the absence of disease though the mucous flows backward against gravity into the back of the throat. Once there it can be swallowed into the stomach where any bacteria and viruses are destroyed.

The air then leaves the nose (or mouth) and enters the trachea, otherwise known as the windpipe. The trachea then splits in two, one for each lung. Like branches on a tree, the bronchi continue to split, getting smaller and smaller. After about 15 generations the bronchi terminate into microscopic bronchioles, which are attached to very tiny air sacs called alveoli. These air sacs are so small that the lung tissue only appears to be solid to the naked eye. In reality, they are only a single cell thick and very membranous. It is here that the oxygen exchange takes place with the equally tiny blood vessels known as capillaries. In fact the capillaries are so small individual blood cells have to squeeze through them single file.

Now how do we use this knowledge in order to maximize your bodies' energy production? The key thing to remember is that your lungs are somewhat triangle shaped with a larger base on the bottom and narrower at the top. In order to maximize the oxygen exchange and therefore your body's energy production you want to ensure that it is the base of your lungs that are constantly being filled with fresh oxygen. As the base of your lungs contain the widest surface area, not to mention that due to gravity blood pools more easily at the bottom, this ensures that the maximum oxygen exchange takes place.

Now that we understand the importance of maximizing the oxygen exchange process we need to look at the three different types of breathing you can perform and how we can use this to our advantage.

The first type of breathing is known as diaphragmatic breathing. The diaphragm is the large muscle located below the lungs that separates the thorax from the abdomen. When it is relaxed this muscle bulges upward in a dome shape which compresses the lungs. When we contract the diaphragm it becomes a flat disc. This expands the lungs from the bottom and allows for the greatest amount of air to enter.

The second type of breathing you can perform is known as chest breathing. This involves the intercostal muscles, which are the muscles that are attached to the ribs. When they are activated the rib cage expands allowing air into the upper and middle sections of the lungs.

The third type of breathing is known as clavicle breathing. This involves pulling the clavicles (collarbone) muscles upwards. It is used to get air into the very top of the lungs.

From what you know now it should be obvious that of these three breathing methods you should endeavor to engage in diaphragmatic breathing at all times. Chest and clavicle breathing should only be used when the body is under severe stress, such as when playing a strenuous sport. Even then, chest and clavicle breathing should only be used in conjunction with diaphragmatic breathing, not replacing it.

Important Note

We are now ready to start exploring various kinds of deep breathing exercises. Before we do though, I want to stress the importance of not taking these exercises lightly. Before you begin any exercise program, including this one, I highly recommend that you talk to your doctor first. This is especially true if you have any form of high blood pressure. As you read through these exercises you will see that many of them involve holding your breath for short periods of time. If you do have high blood pressure, I would recommend that you NOT hold your breath until you talk with your doctor. The act of holding your breath will cause your blood pressure to rise. If this is an issue for you you will need to approach it with extreme caution. As a general rule you should never force any of these exercises. If you are feeling faint or dizzy at anytime simply stop and take a break until the feeling passes. It may take your body some time to get used to breathing properly. Make sure you give it that time by taking it easy.

Basic Diaphragmatic Breathing

Just by paying attention to breathing, you can access new levels of health and relaxation that will benefit every area of your life – Deepak Chopra, M.D.

Now that you know why proper deep breathing is so important for your health and mental well being, we can now start training your body to do it. What follows is a lesson in how to perform basic diaphragmatic breathing along with some variations involving various hand positions and nasal breathing. Always remember that proper diaphragmatic breathing is not meant to be done only at specific times. Rather, you should endeavor to breathe from your diaphragm with deep slow breaths through the day. If you are ever feeling stressed or just a little off take a moment and analyze how you are breathing. By focusing on your breath you will likely feel better in no time.

How to Perform a Diaphragmatic Breath

Improper breathing is a common cause of ill health. Changing your breathing patterns can affect and improve you mentally, emotionally and physically – Andrew Weil, M.D.

Before you attempt your first proper diaphragmatic breath you will want to assume a comfortable deep breathing posture which can mean standing, sitting, or lying flat on the floor. If you are standing or seated try rocking slightly from side to side in order to align your tailbone with the top of your head. You should feel as if the weight of your head is directly above your spinal column. To accomplish this you may need to pull your chin in slightly. Remember that with whatever posture you assume you want your back to be comfortably straight but not rigid. Once you are relaxed perform the following:

1. Begin to breath exclusively through your nose by placing your tongue on the roof of your mouth while keeping your mouth closed.
2. Place your left hand on your chest and your right hand on your abdomen just below your belly button.
3. Begin to inhale through your nose for a count of 5. As you do so visualize your diaphragm pulling down on your lungs to expand them. At the same time use your minds eye to imagine clean, pure air flowing into your nose and filling your lungs.
4. Hold this breath for a count of 7.

5. Exhale through your nose for a count of 8 and repeat. As you exhale imagine that you are expelling toxic gas in some form. I find the image of exhaling black smoke works quite well for me.

As you inhale and exhale pay attention to your hands. If you are performing this deep diaphragmatic breath correctly the hand on your abdomen should always be the first to move, not the one on your chest. Your aim is to always have your lungs fill up with oxygen from the bottom, never the top. Visualizing your breath in some form is very important as well. The incoming breath is the energizing breath; while the outgoing breath will help you relieve tension and stress.

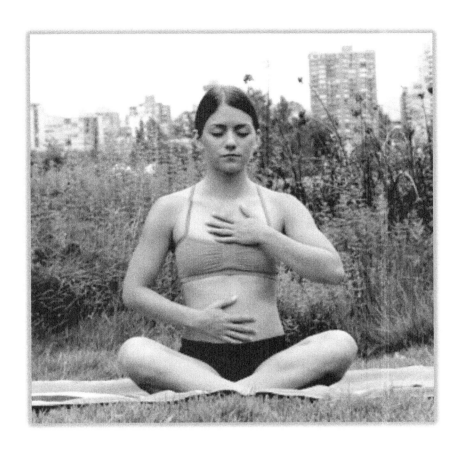

Hand Postures for Deeper Meditation

Breathing is our connection to life, through the body and heart, leading us to a wholeness of being and giving us spirit for living life to its fullest. – S. Hainer, M.S.

Once you are confident you are performing the deep diaphragmatic breath correctly you will want to incorporate some of these hand positions to enhance your practice. In India these are called *Mudras* and they can have a subtle yet powerful affect on the mind/body connection.

Prayer Seal (Anjali Mudra)

To perform this mudra gently put your two palms together with your thumbs placed against your breastbone. By joining your hands together in this manner you are making a physical gesture that you recognize the interconnectedness of all living things. This mudra is thought to be calming as it helps to harmonize the left and right hemispheres of the brain.

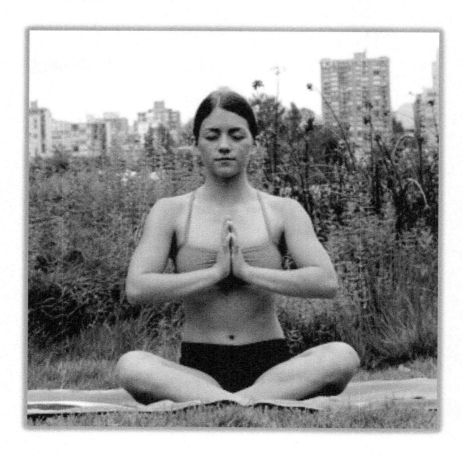

Chin Mudra

To perform this mudra you will want to touch your thumb to your index finger with your palms facing downwards. In many yoga texts the index finger represents the soul and the thumb represents universal consciousness. By bringing your fingers together in this way you are allowing your soul to get in touch with a higher power. Having your palm face down helps to seal in the awareness of this higher consciousness.

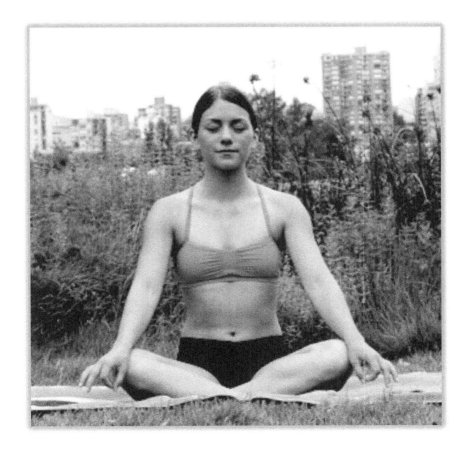

Gyana Mudra

This mudra is similar to the Chin Mudra with the exception that it is performed with the palms facing upward. In yoga texts this helps to calm the mind while sealing in wisdom.

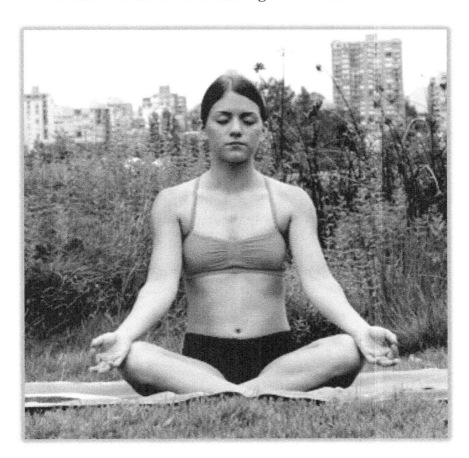

Hakini Mudra

This mudra is said to help with thinking and concentration by aiding in the coordination between the right and left centers of the brain. It can be practiced anywhere at anytime when you feel you need to clear your mind. If you are having difficulty recalling a fact or thought practicing the Hakini Mudra can often help you recall it. To perform the Hakini Mudra do the following:

1. Hold your hands in front of you with your palms facing each other. Do not bring your palms together, however.
2. Touch the fingertips of your right hand with their counterparts on your left.
3. When you perform your diaphragmatic breath inhale through your nose with your tongue against the roof of your mouth.
4. When you exhale through your nose allow your tongue to relax.

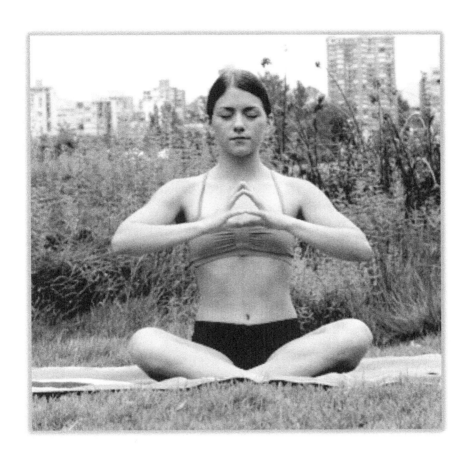

Yoni Mudra

With this mudra you will be creating a downward facing triangle with your hands, which is meant to symbolize the womb as a source of life energy. This mudra will calm your mind and will allow you to relax as you focus on your breath work.

1. Begin with your hands resting just below your navel.
2. Interlock your fingers and spread your hands slightly.
3. Straighten your index fingers so that they are pointed downwards with the tips touching.
4. Touch the tips of your thumbs together and straighten them as well.

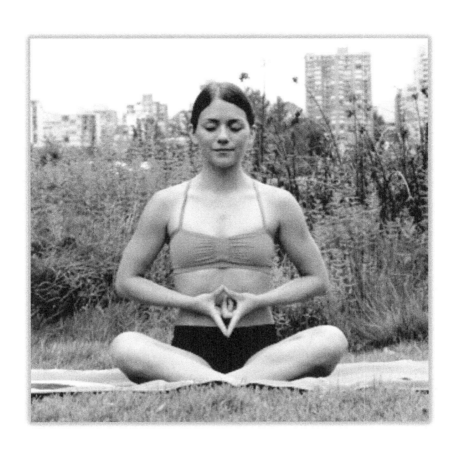

Relaxation Techniques – Nasal Breathing

The natural healing force within you is the greatest force in getting well. – Hippocrates, widely regarded as the father of medicine, 400 B.C.

The final basic diaphragmatic breathing variation we will look at involves alternate nostril breathing. You are likely not aware of this but your body is constantly favoring one nostril over another at all times. This allows one nostril to recharge while its opposite is performing the primary function of purifying the incoming air. To yogis and many other deep breathing practitioners this alternating nostril-breathing pattern actually affects your mind as well. Through thousands of years of practice they have come to believe that the left nostril accesses the right hemisphere of the brain. This is the feminine, cooling side of the brain that is most often associated with creative and dreamy thoughts. Your right nostril is associated with your left, masculine side of your brain. This part of the brain is the analytical, competitive side of your mind. By consciously alternating your nasal breathing patterns during a session of deep meditative breathing you will be able to access and bring balance to both sides of your mind. This will have the effect of calming your mind and nervous system. Once again, by consciously controlling your breath you will be able to gain control and calm your body and mind. This is how you perform this relaxation technique.

1. While performing a session of diaphragmatic breathing use your right thumb to close off your right nostril.
2. Inhale slowly through your left nostril with a deep diaphragmatic breath for a count of 5.
3. Hold your breath for a count of 7.
4. Close your left nostril with your ring finger and release the thumb off your right nostril.
5. Exhale through your right nostril, completely emptying your lungs, for a count of 8.
6. Inhale slowly through your right nostril for a count of 5.
7. Hold your breath for a count of 7. As you do so release your left nostril and close your right with your thumb.
8. Breathe out through your left nostril for a count of 8.

This counts as one complete round of nasal breathing. I suggest you start slowly by performing one or two rounds at first and increasing that over time. Once again if you have any kind of issues with high blood pressure do not hold your breath. You may find at times that one of your nostrils is so blocked that you cannot breathe any air out of it. Do not let this concern you. This simply means that you have caught your body at the height of it nostril-cleaning cycle. In these situations I suggest you simply wait for a bit until your nostril clears up enough to perform deep nasal breaths. Remember, deep breathing should always be a relaxing and calming experience. Never force it.

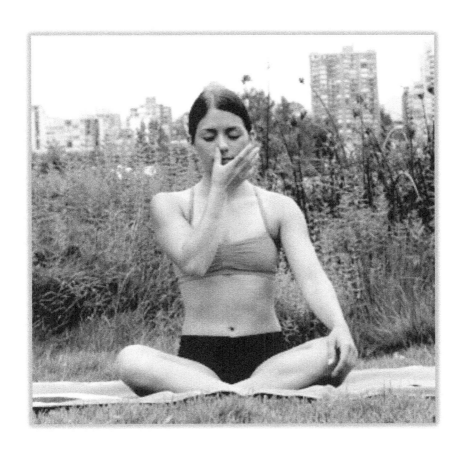

Breathing Exercises for Specific Conditions

Life is in the breath. He who half breathes, half lives! – Old Proverb

The basic full diaphragmatic breath, along with the mudra and nasal breathing variations, are really all you need to improve your breathing. Simply practicing them in some form for 5 to 10 minutes a day will do wonders for your health and happiness. There are countless varieties of deep breathing exercises out there, however. What follows are a few I have come across that have helped others with various conditions. You can either use them as a supplement to the basic diaphragmatic breath or perform them by themselves anytime throughout the day. It's up to you.

Deep Breathing for Insomnia

He who can't find time for exercise will have time for illness. – Lord Derby

Millions of people worldwide suffer from insomnia and poor sleep. To help alleviate this condition I would recommend you first have a cold shower right before you go to bed. How cold? As cold as you can handle. I suggest you start with a mildly cold shower and gradually lower the temperature over the course of a five-minute period. This has the effect of cooling your body and preparing it for sleep. Once you have finished with your cold shower go lie down in a properly ventilated room and try performing one of these two deep breathing exercises.

Deep Breathing for Insomnia Variation #1

1. Begin by lying flat on your back in your bed with your hands by your sides, palms down.
2. Close your eyes. Begin to inhale through your nose as you simultaneously begin to raise your arms up over your head.
3. Continue to inhale, completely filling your lungs, until your arms are straight above your head on the ground. For every inhale you take your arms should move like this in a 180 degree fashion.
4. Hold this breath for a count of 8 to 10 seconds.

5. Begin to exhale slowly out of your nose as you raise your arms and return them to the starting position. You should time it so that your arms come to rest beside you just as you finish your exhale.
6. Repeat this exercise 4 to 10 times or until you start to become drowsy.

At this point you should be feeling very relaxed. You may want to drift off to sleep my listening to some gentle music or a podcast of some kind. You'll be asleep in no time.

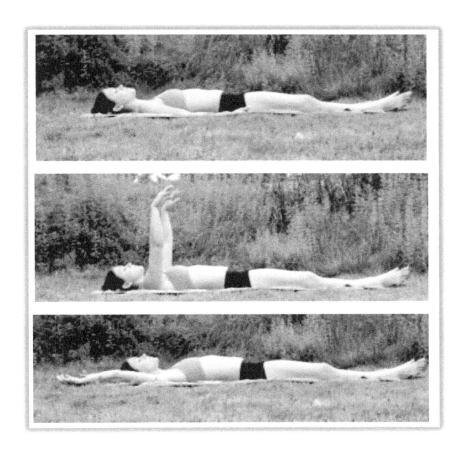

Deep Breathing for Insomnia Variation
#2

1. Get into bed and lie flat on your back.
2. Close your eyes and take a deep breath in through your nose as you slowly count to 5.
3. As you breathe in imagine you can see the air as it flows through your nose and into your lungs.
4. Hold this breath for a count of 4.
5. Exhale your lungs completely by breathing out through your nose for a count of 8.
6. Repeat this breathing technique 6 to 10 more times or until you start to feel drowsy.

Taking a cold shower before you perform this mediation and listening to something soothing afterwards works well for this relaxation technique too.

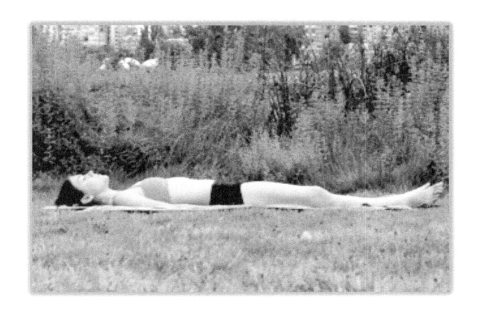

Anti-aging Breathing Exercises

We must always change, renew, rejuvenate ourselves; otherwise, we harden. – Johann W. Goethe

As we age the breathing capacity of our lungs and the flexibility of our rib cage tends to diminish. These breathing exercises are designed to ameliorate these tendencies if not out right reverse them.

Anti-aging Breathing Exercise #1

This breathing exercise is meant to increase your lungs capacity to store air.

1. Begin by bending forward and placing the palms of your hands on your bent knees. Exhale all of the air from your lungs through your nose.
2. Begin to inhale through your nose as you slowly start to stand up straight.
3. As you continue to stand up straight raise both of your arms over your head until your lungs are completely filled with air.
4. Hold your breath for a count of 8 seconds with your arms above your head.
5. Begin to exhale through your nose as you bend over at the waist and return to the starting position.
6. Repeat this movement 2 or 3 more times.

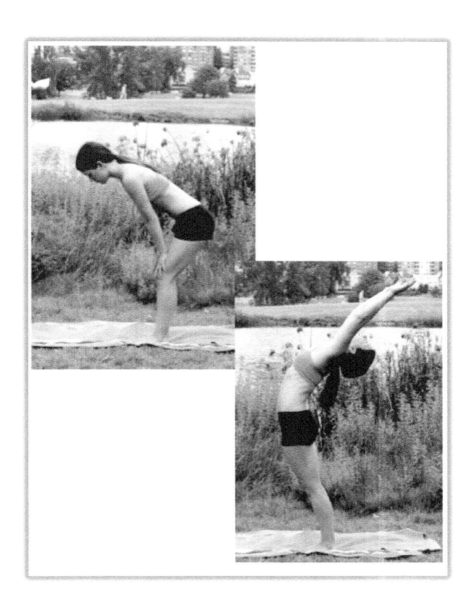

Anti-Aging Breathing Exercise #2

The aim of this breathing exercise is to help keep your rib cage flexible so that it can expand easily when you breathe.

1. Begin by standing with your arms by your sides. Exhale all of the air from your lungs through your nose.
2. Slowly inhale through your nose so that you completely fill your lungs.
3. Hold your breath while placing your palms on your hips with your pinkie fingers touching other on your back. Now pull your elbows back as far as you can while still holding your breath. Try to hold this position for a count of 10.
4. Slowly exhale through your nose as you lower your arms back by your sides.
5. Repeat this breathing exercise 2 or 3 more times.

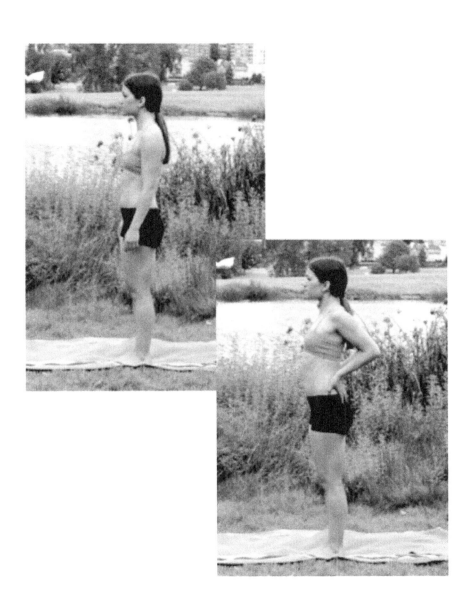

Deep Breathing Exercises for Asthma

Diaphragmatic breathing is beneficial as it enhances circulatory function and relaxes the muscles of ribs, chest and stomach. – Susan Smith Jones, Ph. D.

Asthma is an all to common condition in which a person's airways become constricted, making breathing difficult. All of the deep breathing exercises found in this book can help with this condition. What follows are some deep breathing exercises that some have found to be particularly effective. However do not limit yourself to them if you are an asthma suffer. You may want to start here but as your breathing gets stronger don't limit yourself to them. Listen to your body and how it feels. You may find that some other breathing exercise helps you to get to a new level of healthy living and relaxed breathing.

Asthma Treatment #1 – Chest Expander

This breathing exercise will help you gain control over your inhalation and exhalation while expanding your chest. As you get stronger you can increase the amount of time you hold your breath. Just remember to only hold your breath to the point where you are comfortable. Never force yourself to hold your breath to the point where you feel faint or ill. Go slowly and use common sense.

1. Begin with your arms straight out in front of you at shoulder level. Your palms should be facing each other.
2. Inhale through your nose for a count of 4 as your move your arms as far back as possible, which will help you expand your chest. As you do so imagine that you have a "life force" existing between your palms. You can imagine it anyway you want, but I like to see it as a ball of vibrant, cracking energy. As you separate your palms imagine this ball of energy growing and becoming more powerful. This visualization technique will help your mind focus to get the most out of your breathing and will really help energize you. The energy ball you are seeing in your minds eye is a representation of what you are actually doing in your lungs.
3. Hold your breath for a count of 4.
4. Exhale through your nose for a count of 4 as you bring your palms back together (shrinking the energy ball as you do so).

46

5. Perform this exercise for a minimum of
   4 to 6 times or as long as you like.

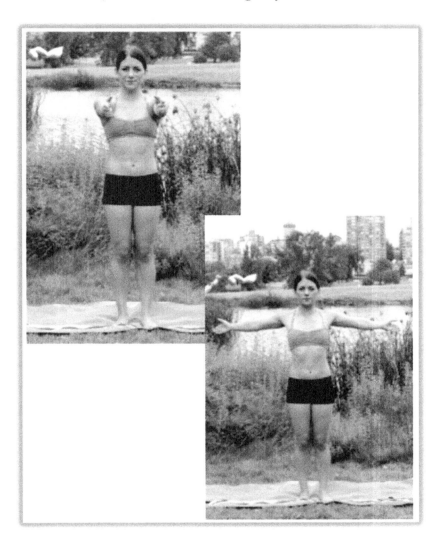

Asthma Treatment #2 – Chest Extender

This breathing exercise is similar to asthma treatment #1 except we will be working on extending and expanding your chest forward. Once again as you get stronger you can work on holding your breath for longer periods of time.

1. Begin with your feet together and your palms facing each other near your chest.
2. As you inhale your breath through your nose for a count of 4 extend your arms forward away from your chest. You should finish with your palms facing forward at shoulder level.
3. Hold your breath for another count of 4.
4. Exhale through your nose for a count of 4 as you bring your arms back to the starting position.
5. Repeat this breathing exercise 4 to 6 times.

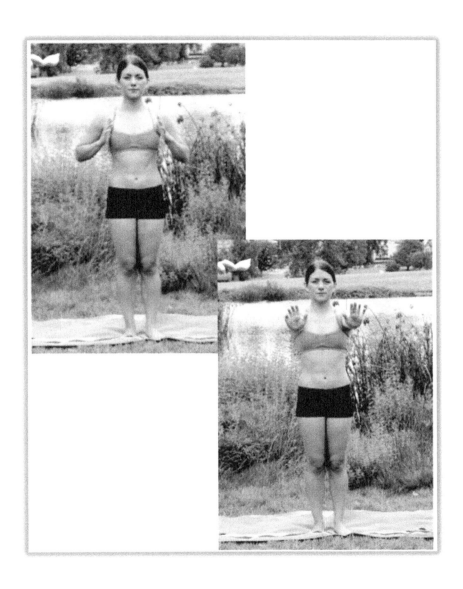

Asthma Treatment #3 – Candle Blowing

With this breathing exercise you will be purposely breathing out through your mouth instead of your nose for once. The reason for this is that it allows you to put gentle pressure on the lungs, which will work your diaphragm and other abdominal muscles.

1. Begin with your feet shoulder width apart and your hands on your hips just below your rib cage.
2. Inhale through your nose for a count of 4, completely filling your lungs.
3. Hold your breath for a count of 2.
4. Exhale slowly and steadily through your mouth. Purse your lips, almost like you're blowing out a candle. It should take you between 8 and 10 counts to completely exhale all of the air from your lungs.
5. Perform this exercise between 2 and 4 times.

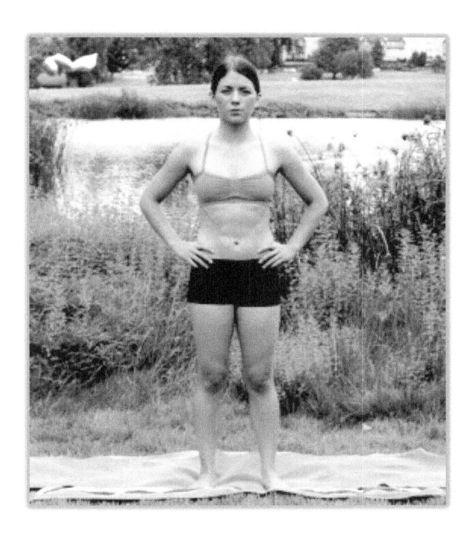

Breathing Exercises for Panic Attacks and Anxiety Relief

The quality of breath should be deep, graceful, easy and efficient. – Kenneth Cohen

As I have already noted, your emotional state affects your breath. When you are experiencing anxiety, stress or panic your breath typically becomes shallow and quick. When you are aware of this, however, you can use your breath to reverse this process and gain control over your emotions. The next time you are experiencing a panic attack or some form of anxiety try the following:

1. First of all, use the thumb and forefinger of one hand to firmly massage the skin between the thumb and forefinger of the opposite hand. This is a form of self-acupressure that will help ease a nervous stomach. This technique by itself can also be helpful with motion sickness.
2. As you continue to massage your hands, concentrate on your breath. Breathe in deeply through your nose for a count of 4.
3. Hold your breath for a count of 4 as you roll your shoulders forward and backward a couple of times.
4. Exhale through your nose for a count of 4. Imagine you are blowing all of the stress and tension from your body as you do so.

5. With your lungs empty, don't breathe in for a few seconds. Instead, force your stomach muscles in and out 4 times.
6. Breathe in again through your nose for a count of 4, and repeat this process 5 times. When you are done you should feel more relaxed and peaceful.

Note that this exercise can be done either sitting or standing.

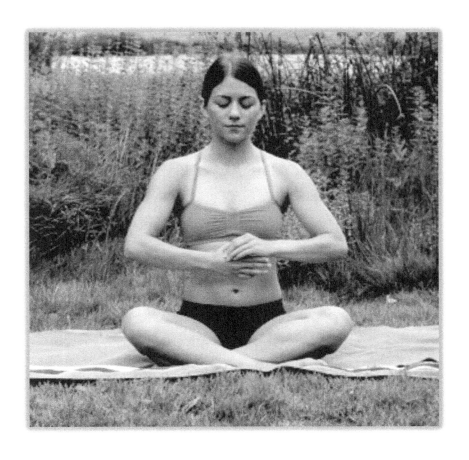

A Breathing Exercise for Fatigue

He who breathes the most air, lives the better life. – Elizabeth Barrett Browning

Adenosine Triphosphate (or ATP for short) is a by-product of breathing that helps to regulate physical action and mood. During the day you may experience dips in your ATP levels, which can result in fatigue, aches and pain. This one breath meditation can help to reverse falling ATP levels and can be done anywhere at anytime.

1. Sit in a comfortable chair with your back straight and your shoulders relaxed.
2. Close your eyes and inhale through your nose as slowly and deeply as you can. Imagine your body filling up with energizing oxygen from the bottom of your lungs to the top.
3. Hold your breath for a moment and then start to exhale through your nose as slowly as you can. Imagine you are releasing all of the tension and fatigue from your body.

This one-minute refreshing breath can be done at home, during a workout, or anytime you need a quick boost of energy. It will refresh and restore your body, mind and soul all at once. Give it a try and see for yourself.

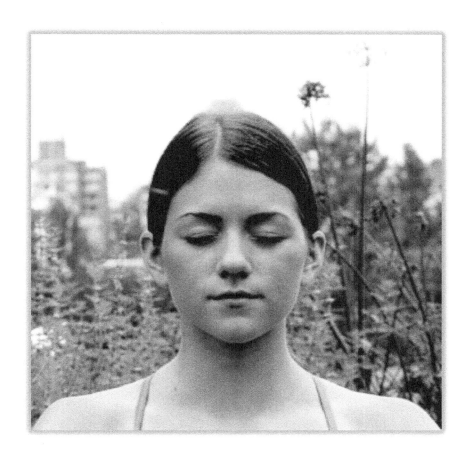

Breathing Exercises for Happiness

God gave His creatures light and air and water open to the skies; Man locks himself in a stifling lair and wonders why his brother dies.
– Oliver W. Holmes, Associate Justice to U.S. Supreme Court, 1902-1932

Aside from the myriad of other benefits already mentioned deep breathing can have the effect of instilling in the practitioner a sense of well being and happiness. By itself deep diaphragmatic breathing can help lift feelings of depression and improve your mood. Although all deep-breathing exercises can have this effect the following two excel at it. Please note though that when performing these exercises for the first time you may not be able to hold your breath for the full count at first. If you experience any discomfort at all, such as dizziness, return to the standing position immediately and relax until the feeling passes. As always go slowly and use common sense.

The Cleansing Breath

This breathing exercise will help to energize you while purging your body of negative emotions.

1. Begin by standing with your feet comfortably apart and your hands by your sides.
2. Inhale through your nose as you raise your arms above your head while bending your back backward. Bend as far back as you can comfortably while looking at the sky until your lungs are completely filled with air.
3. Hold your breath in this position for 4 to 5 seconds.
4. Exhale through your nose as you bend forward at the waist. Keep your knees slightly bent as you do so. When you have bent forward as far as you can, make an effort to really suck your stomach in in order to expel every last bit of air possible.
5. Begin to inhale through your nose as you slowly start to stand up again, raising your hands above your head.
6. Repeat this motion 5 times.

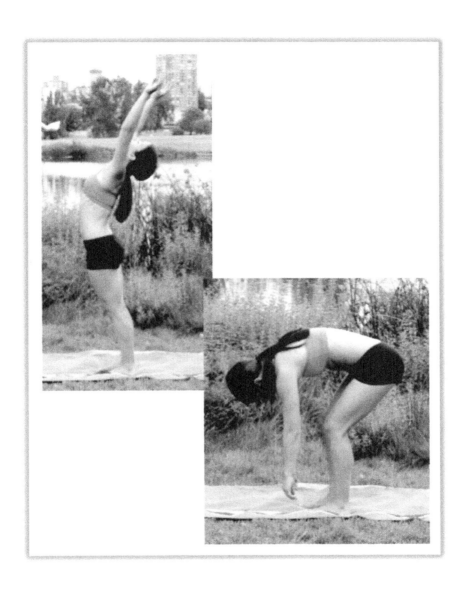

The Happiness Breath

The physical motion of the happiness breath is very similar to the cleansing breath. The difference between the two exercises is in how long and when you hold the breath. When done properly the happiness breath is excellent at recharging your brain while helping to clean out your skull cavities (such as your sinuses, ears and nose).

1. Just like the cleansing breath, begin by standing with your feet comfortably apart and your hands by your sides.
2. Inhale through your nose as you raise your arms above your head while bending your back backward. Bend as far back as you can comfortably while looking at the sky until your lungs are completely filled with air.
3. Hold your breath as you bend forward at the waist. Keep your knees slightly bent as you do so. Bend forward as far as you can and attempt to continue to hold your breath for a count of 10.
4. Continue to hold your breath as you return to the standing position with your hands above your head.
5. Bend forward again as you now exhale all of the breath through your nose.
6. Inhale through your nose as you slowly start to stand up again, raising your hands above your head.
7. Repeat this motion 5 times.

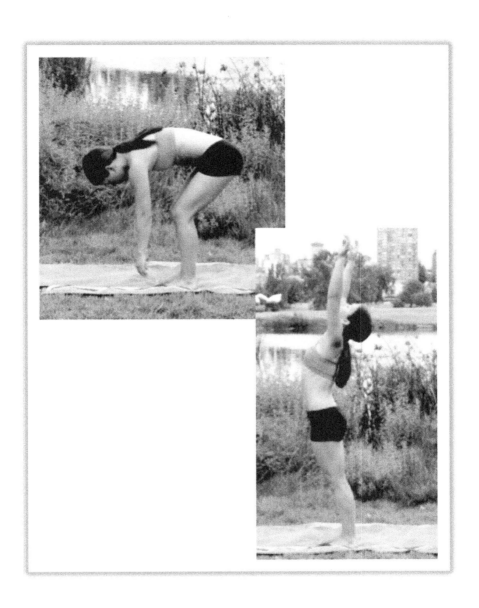

Breathing Exercises for Healthy Living and Energy

It is exercise alone that supports the spirits, and keeps the mind in vigor. -Marcus Tullius Cicero

Reach for the Sky

1. Begin by standing with your feet comfortably together and your hands on your shoulders.
2. As you begin to inhale through your nose start to raise your hands upwards with the palms down. You should time the inhale with the raising motion of your hands so that your lungs are completely filled with oxygen when your arms are fully extended.
3. Exhale through your nose as you lower your hands back to your shoulders. Your lungs should be completely empty by the time your hands touch your shoulders.
4. Repeat this motion 10 times.

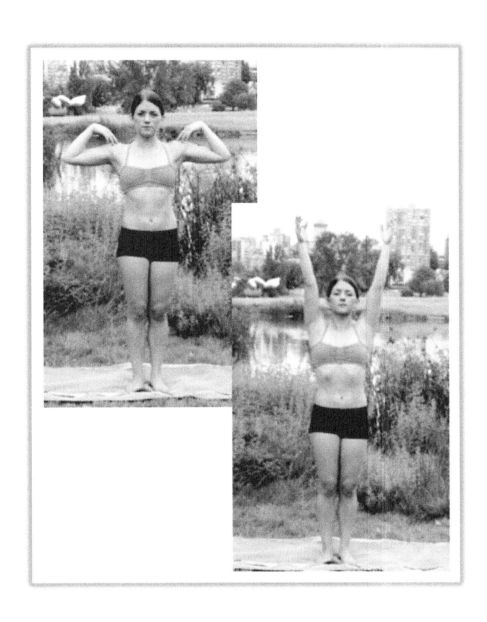

Hands Forward

1. Begin by standing with your feet comfortably together and your hands on your shoulders. This is the starting position.
2. As you begin to inhale through your nose extend your hands straight out in front of you with your palms facing forward. Your lungs should be completely filled with oxygen by the time your arms reach the point of maximum extension.
3. Exhale through your nose as you return your hands to the starting position. Your lungs should be completely empty by the time your hands reach your shoulders.
4. Repeat this motion 10 times.

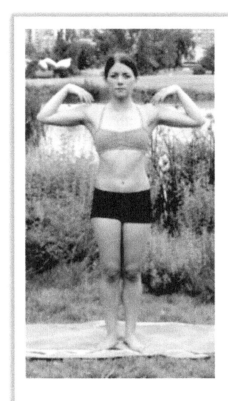

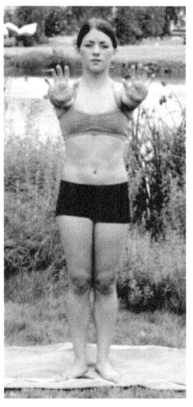

Hands to the Side

1. Begin by standing with your feet comfortably together and your hands on your shoulders. This is the starting position.
2. As you begin to inhale through your nose extend your hands to either side with your palms facing outward. Your lungs should be completely filled with oxygen when your arms reach the point of maximum extension.
3. Exhale through your nose as you return your hands to the starting position. Your lungs should be completely empty by the time your hands reach your shoulders.
4. Repeat this motion 10 times.

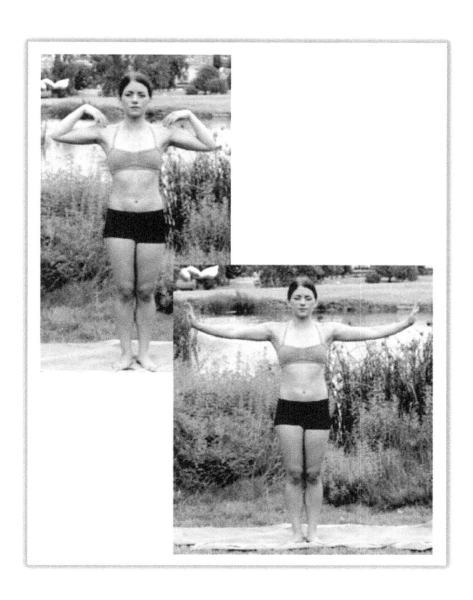

Healthy Living Arm Crosses

This exercise is adapted from a breathing exercise found in China. Known as Qi Gong (Chi King) the motion of this exercise, particularly the crossing of the arms, promotes internal energy, happiness and healthy living.

1. Begin by bending forward at the waist with your arms crossed just below the elbows in front of you with your palms down. This is the starting position.
2. Inhale through your nose as you straighten your spine and then bend backwards. As you do so, bring your arms to your sides with the palms upward and look up towards the sky as you completely fill your lungs.
3. Exhale through your nose as you return. Bend forward again and return your arms to the starting position.
4. Repeat this motion 10 times.

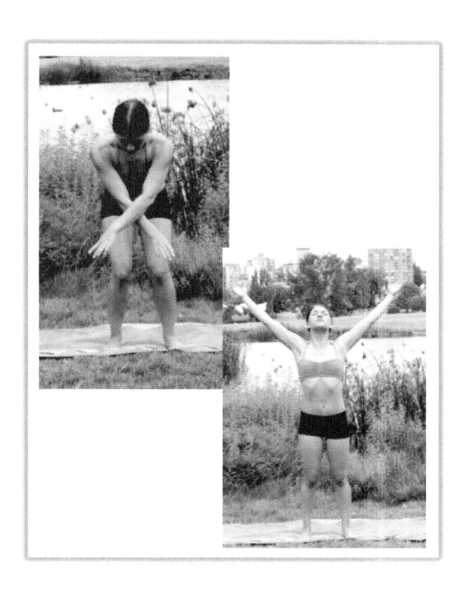

Deep Breathing FAQ

I've read many exercise and fitness books and they often recommend breathing in through the nose and out through the mouth. You seem to emphasize breathing in and out through the nose exclusively. Why is this?

The nose is designed by nature to be the primary method by which we breathe. There are a variety of systems in the nose designed to purify the air before they reach the lungs. However the nose is also meant to expel air as well. The air purifying systems within your nose actually require air to flow out of the nose to operate at peak efficiency, primarily because it helps to expel dust and debris. Breathing out through your mouth prevents this from happening.

I know I should breathe through my nose, but I simply find it easier to breathe through my mouth.

A lot of people think this way, but it's really just a case of getting used to breathing through your nose. I've also read studies that it actually costs the body 50% more in energy when we breathe in through the mouth as opposed to the nose. The reason for this is that air received via the mouth has not been optimized to be absorbed by the lungs. This is inefficient and costs your body more energy in the long run.

I find that my mind wanders during my mediation and breathing sessions. What can I do?

First of all don't concern yourself with this. Particularly in the beginning it is not uncommon for beginners to have trouble concentrating. Our minds are used to constantly working throughout the day. Switching gears and allowing our minds to rest is actually a lot harder than you might think. The first thing I would recommend doing is to stop being so hard on yourself and worrying about how active your mind is. When thoughts come into your mind, whether positive or negative, acknowledge them and let them pass without comment. Simply focus on your breath and let these thoughts pass like clouds in the sky. With time you will find your mind calming. It does take time, but you can do it.

How can I be sure that I am performing these deep breathing and relaxation techniques correctly?

So long as your abdomen moves up or out as you inhale and contracts or moves inward as you exhale you're on the right track. The key is to always breath from the base of you lungs (deep breathing) as opposed to the top (shallow breathing), which most people do.

I think all of this talk about "pranayama", "chi gong", meditation and yoga relaxation techniques are a bunch of new age hooey.

That's not really a question, but you're more than entitled to your opinion. The truth of the matter is that you don't have to believe in the more spiritual aspects of these exercises in order to get positive benefits from them. I urge you to keep an open mind and give the breathing exercises a try just like you would with anything else. I'm confident you'll find one or two that will benefit you.

I often feel light headed after I've completed a deep breathing session. Why is this?

A lightheaded feeling or even excessive yawning is not uncommon when you start practicing deep diaphragmatic breathing. Most likely it is an indication that your body has become accustomed to shallow breathing and is not used to this much oxygen coursing through it. You may want to try breathing a little less deeply for a few sessions in order to give your body time to adapt. Work on taking deeper breaths as the light headed feelings recede and you feel more comfortable.

Can I perform my deep breathing practice anywhere?

Yes, you can. That is one of the great things about breathing exercises. If you are at work or standing in line you can take a moment, focus on your breath, and reap the benefits. Having said that however you would likely greatly benefit by setting aside a dedicated time (10 minutes?) to focus on your breathing practice. All you need is a quiet, well-ventilated room (or outside, weather permitting) that is free of distractions (turn your cell phone off). With time I'm sure that you'll find that regular practice in such a quiet space will benefit you immensely.

Further Reading

If you enjoyed my book you will likely find these books useful as well:

52 Small Changes: One Year to a Happier, Healthier You by Brett Blumenthal

The Stress Free You: How to Live Stress Free and Feel Great Everyday, Starting Today by Elizabeth O'Brien

Super Brain: Unleashing the Explosive Power of Your Mind to Maximize Health, Happiness, and Spiritual Well-Being by Rudolph Tanzi and Deepak Chopra

How to Meditate: A Practical Guide to Making Friends with Your Mind by Perma Chodron

Happiness: A Guide to Developing Life's Most Important Skill by Matthieu Ricard

Wherever You Go, There You Are: Mindfulness Meditation in Everyday Life by Jon Kabat-Zinn

Meditation for Warriors by Loren W. Christensen

Buddha's Brain: The Practical Neuroscience of Happiness, Love, and Wisdom by Rick Hanson

About the Author

Anthony Anholt has been interested and involved in athletics and fitness for his entire life. His specialty is "gymless" workouts, or exercise systems that do not require any kind of special equipment. He is also interested in enhancing performance in all sports, but particularly basketball. This is his fourth book.

About the Model

Dana Sorensen is a Vancouver based fitness instructor, performer and dancer. She can be contacted for modeling work here: http://www.modelmayhem.com/1709968

One Last Thing

You've now reached the end of the book and I hope you find it useful in building a better you. If you did find it useful I would very much appreciate it if you could take 5 minutes and write a short review for it on Amazon or wherever you purchased it. Even a couple of sentences would be immensely helpful to me. Regardless I want to thank-you once again for purchasing my book and I wish you all the best in the future.

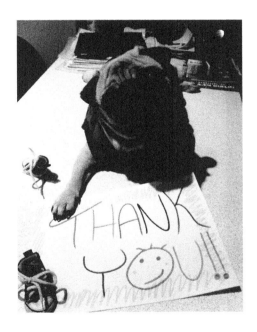

Made in the USA
Monee, IL
15 February 2022

91301538R00046